Table of Contents

Introduction: Society of Urologic Nurses and Associates 2
SUNA's Mission Statement 2
SUNA's Vision 2
Recognition of the Specialty 2
Approval of the Scope of Practice 3
Acknowledgment of the Standards of Practice 3
Scope and Standards Workgroup Members (2010-2012) 3
Reviewers and Contributors 3
Scope of Urologic Nursing Practice 5
    Definition of Urologic Nursing 5
    Practice Population/Environment 6
    Differentiation of Registered Nurse and Advanced Practice Registered Nurse Roles
    In Urologic Nursing 8
    Professional Education and Development for Registered Nurses and Advanced Practice
    Registered Nurses 10
    Evolution of Urologic Nursing Practice and SUNA 11
    Current Issues and Trends in Health Care Affecting Urologic Nursing 13
    Summary 18
Standards of Urologic Nursing Practice 20
    Standard 1: Assessment 20
    Standard 2: Diagnosis 21
    Standard 3: Outcomes Identification 22
    Standard 4: Planning 23
    Standard 5: Implementation 24
    Standard 5a: Coordination of Care 25
    Standard 5b: Health Teaching and Health Promotion 25
    Standard 5c: Consultation 26
    Standard 5d: Prescriptive Authority and Treatment 26
    Standard 6: Evaluation 27
Standards of Professional Performance 28
    Standard 7: Ethics 28
    Standard 8: Education 29
    Standard 9: Evidence-Based Practice and Research 29
    Standard 10: Quality of Practice 30
    Standard 11: Communication 31
    Standard 12: Leadership 32
    Standard 13: Collaboration 33
    Standard 14: Professional Practice Evaluation 33
    Standard 15: Resource Utilization 34
    Standard 16: Environmental Health 35
References 36

INTRODUCTION

Society of Urologic Nurses and Associates

The Society of Urologic Nurses and Associates (SUNA) is a non-profit, national and international professional membership association of urologic nurses and associates[1] with a common goal of advancing the profession of urologic care through standards of excellence. SUNA is a specialty organization that supports culturally appropriate nursing care of patients across the lifespan. SUNA is collectively responsible for setting forth the scope of practice for both the urologic registered nurse (RN) and advanced practice registered nurse (APRN) with the understanding that the American Nurses Association (ANA) establishes the scope of practice for all levels of professional nursing practice and provides the foundation for this document. The scope of urologic nursing is dynamic and flexible. Urologic nursing represents a system, which is an ever-broadening practice, expanding as required by a changing health care system in a manner commensurate with its underlying theoretical framework, knowledge base, and professional and legal delineation.

SUNA provides a variety of opportunities for participation at the local, state, national, and international levels. The local level within the national arena includes local chapters, task forces, and special interest groups (SIGs) in seven major subspecialty areas. Urologic nurses care for patients across the lifespan, providing guidance and treatment for a variety of urologic diseases and concerns. Recognizing the need to advance urologic nursing practice and create a continuum of knowledge, the SUNA Board of Directors approved the formation of the SUNA Foundation in 2006. The foundation supports members in their pursuit of urologic nursing research, specialized training in urologic care, and educational programs by funding scholarships. To recognize how valuable urologic nurses and associates are to the health care system and to their patients, SUNA established *Urology Nurses and Associates Week,* which is promoted and celebrated each year, November 1-7.

Mission

As a professional community of urologic nurses and associates, SUNA is committed to enriching the professional lives of our members and improving the health of our patients and their families, through education, research, and evidence-based clinical practice.

Vision

A dynamic, varied and robust organization, SUNA is recognized by medical professionals, patients, their families, and the public as the nursing authority on collaborative, compassionate, and culturally competent urologic care.

Recognition of the Specialty

The American Nurses Association recognizes urologic nursing as a nursing specialty.

---

[1] SUNA member associates include technicians, medical assistants, physician's assistants, educators, physicians, physical therapists, students, industry representatives, and other urologic health care professionals.

Approval of the Scope of Practice

The American Nurses Association has approved the Urologic Nursing Scope and Standards of Practice as defined herein. Approval is valid for five (5) years from the first date of publication of this document or until a new scope and standards of practice has been approved, whichever occurs first.

Acknowledgment of the Standards of Practice

The American Nurses Association acknowledges the Urologic Nursing Scope and Standards of Practice, as set forth herein. Acknowledgment is valid for five (5) years from the first date of publication of this document or until new standards of practice have been published, whichever occurs first.

Scope and Standards Workgroup Members (2010-2012)

Debbie Hensley, BSN, RN, CURN, *Chair*
Amy Driscoll, BSN, CURN, CCCN, *Co-Chair*
Christine Bradway, PhD, GNP-BC, FAAN
Jean F. Wyman, PhD, GNP-BC, FAAN
Phyllis Sheldon, MS, RN, CNS-BC, CUCNS
Gwen Hooper, PhD, APRN, CUNP
Angela Joseph, MSN, CNS, CURN

Reviewers

APN Competency Task Force
Phyllis A. Matthews, MS, ANP-BC, CUNP
Sally S. Russell, MN, CMSRN

Contributors

Barbara Broome, PhD, RN, FAAN
Diane K. Newman, DNP, ANP-BC, FAAN

SCOPE OF UROLOGIC NURSING PRACTICE

This document is based on the American Nurses Association (ANA, 2010a) *Nursing: Scope and Standards of Practice, 2nd Edition,* document. The profession of nursing has one scope of practice that encompasses the full range of nursing practice. Registered nurses (RNs) practicing in the United States have three professional resources that inform practice and decision-making. The *Code of Ethics for Nurses with Interpretive Statements* (ANA, 2001) lists nine succinct provisions that establish the ethical framework for registered nurses across all roles, levels, and settings. Second, *Nursing's Social Policy Statement: The Essence of the Profession* (ANA, 2010b), conceptualizes nursing practice, describes the social context of nursing, and provides the definition of nursing. Finally, *Nursing: Scope and Standards of Practice, 2nd Edition* (ANA, 2010a), outlines the expectations of the professional role of the registered nurse, and presents the scope of practice statement and standards of professional nursing practice and accompanying competencies.

Definition of Urologic Nursing

Urologic nursing is the specialized practice of professional nursing that focuses on assisting the health care consumer in regaining and/or maintaining urologic health as well as preventing co-morbid physical and/or psychological illness associated with urologic conditions. This involves provision of individualized, holistic, and evidence-based care for patients with urologic needs. Urologic nursing deals with diseases of the male and female genitourinary tract and reproductive organs. Urologic nurses perform focused health exams and educate patients on how to best maintain genitourinary health that could significantly impact their quality of life. Throughout this document, the terms *health care consumer* and *patient* will be used interchangeably. The term *family* relates to family members of origin or significant others identified by the health care consumer.

Urologic nursing primarily concentrates on urine transport, storage, and expulsion functions, in contrast to nephrology nursing which emphasizes care of individuals with kidney disease. Urologic nursing is based on a thorough understanding of the structure and function of the urinary system from the nephron (the functional unit of the kidney) to the urethral meatus. The urologic nurse also applies knowledge of the anatomy, physiology, and embryonic development of the male and female genitourinary system to care for patients with disorders of the genitalia and sexual function.

Urologic nurses utilize the nursing process of assessment, diagnosis, outcomes identification, planning, implementation, and evaluation, and work collaboratively with other members of the health care team. Urologic nurses are patient advocates ensuring patient safety and quality of life. Due to a variety of sensitive issues related to genitourinary disorders, caring, empathy, respect, compassion, support, and acceptance are essential to the role of the urologic registered nurse.

Urologic nurses are self-motivated, self-directed, lifelong learners, recognizing the need to: (1) participate in continuing education and professional development to maintain competence; (2) actively conduct and/or collaborate in clinical research projects; (3) utilize current evidence-based practice guidelines to standardize care; (4) read, review, and participate in discussions of professional literature; (5) maintain ongoing collaborative efforts with other members of the health care team; (6) share unique knowledge and skills with other members of the health care team; and (7) seek specialty certification by the Certification Board for Urologic Nurses and Associates (CBUNA). The depth and breadth in which individual RNs engage in the total scope of urologic nursing practice is dependent upon their education, experience, role, and the type of population they serve.

Urologic nurses play an important role in promoting, facilitating, and supporting urologic health by raising public and professional awareness locally, nationally, as well as worldwide. Many urologic nurses volunteer their time and passions to facilitate various monthly support groups for patients with prostate or bladder cancer and interstitial cystitis. Support groups can offer information and help to patients, family members, and significant others to better understand their diagnosis and treatments as well as provide coping skills to better handle health challenges. Urologic nurses across the United States annually participate in World Continence Week to promote awareness about incontinence and related issues, in prostate cancer awareness events, and in Bladder Health Week.

Urologic nursing is a unique nursing specialty that addresses the needs of individuals with urological health care concerns due to injury, aging, cancer, neurological, genetic, reproductive, and medical illnesses. The unique expertise of the urologic nurse is consistently sought out and valued by members of the urology team, the health care community, and the lay community at large. Urologic nurses possess a passion for knowledge, a drive for creativity and innovation, and a sense of mission in caring for the public they serve.

Practice Population/Environment

Urologic nurses practice in a wide range of settings with patients across the lifespan, caring for pediatric, adult, and elderly clients. Knowledge of development and aging changes are essential to help differentiate interactions with acute and chronic disease. Urologic problems may be, but often are not "stand-alone" issues, meaning that the urologic complaint is secondary to a chronic, systemic illness. This requires urologic professionals to have an understanding of chronic illness, such as diabetes or cardiovascular disease. Collaboration with health care professionals in other disciplines is essential. Telephone triage and consultation are becoming increasingly important tools for urologic nurses as they provide education and a continuum of care to health care consumers. The scope of practice for urologic nursing is broad and challenging; spanning sub-specialties such as oncology, neurology, male infertility, male and female sexual dysfunction, voiding dysfunction, kidney stones, trauma, geriatrics, and pediatrics.

The pediatric population includes infants, children, and adolescents experiencing congenital anomalies and neoplasms, urinary tract infections and/or obstructions, inter-sex disorders, voiding disorders/dysfunctions such as primary enuresis (bedwetting), or disease and/or trauma of the genitourinary tract. Pediatric urologic nurses possess the skills to assess the special needs of the pediatric population and their families, and to use a multidisciplinary health care team approach to coordinate a program of care and support in dealing with such specialized urologic disorders, neoplasms, and continence challenges.

Congenital anomalies are also encountered by urologic nurses caring for adult patients. These anomalies can be clinically relevant when they compromise genitourinary function or affect organ development later in life (Gray & Moore, 2009), emphasizing the importance of a focused history and physical examination to uncover significant information needed for the most effective treatment plans. Although these congenital defects influence urologic management, they may not compromise the primary complaint or disorder leading the individual to seek care (Gray & Moore, 2009).

Urologic nurses play a key role in counseling health care consumers and families about genitourinary cancer risk factors, prevention and/or early detection, diagnosis, and treatment options. Genitourinary cancers in adult males are an important aspect of urologic nursing. One in six men is at risk of developing prostate cancer in their lifetime, making prostate cancer the leading cause of new cancer cases in men. Other common genitourinary cancers that affect both adult men and women involve the urinary bladder, kidney, and the renal pelvis.

Geriatric urologic nurses work with older patients experiencing age-related changes of the genitourinary system (incontinence, infections, voiding dysfunction, sexual health issues, and cancers). The field of geriatric urology is growing in response to the aging United States population. Urologic nurses have responded by creating continence programs specific to the long-term care setting, and expanding their role in the area of urogynecology, which in part deals with age-related changes to the female genital tract.

Hospital-based urologic nurses work on inpatient multi-specialty or medical-surgical units, or on a urology-specific inpatient unit. They provide direct care for patients who have undergone urologic procedures (prostate, renal, uro-oncological, or genitourinary surgery), using their specialty training to devise and implement an appropriate plan of care. Additionally, in the hospital setting urologic nurses provide surgical assistance in the operating room or work as specialty consultants or collaborators for urologic issues such as urinary catheter management, continence concerns, patient education development, or urologic conditions which arise secondary to another health concern. Urologic nurses collaborate and consult with wound, ostomy, and continence nurse colleagues preoperatively, when preparing patients for surgical procedures and in the postoperative setting regarding stoma care or other continence care issues involving skin and wound care. Physical therapist colleagues are consulted regarding pelvic floor muscle rehabilitation in both children and adults for dysfunctional voiding and incontinence disorders.

Urologic nurses in outpatient clinical settings provide care in stand-alone offices, large multi-specialty practice sites, and hospital and university-based outpatient clinics. Such clinics are either general urologic practices, urogynecological practices, or have a sub-specialty focus such as urologic cancers (prostate, bladder, renal, testicular), sexual health (male or female sexual dysfunction, gender assignment, and fertility issues), continence management, genitourinary infections, stone disease, other urinary obstructions, trauma, pediatrics, or geriatrics. Urologic nurses perform urodynamic studies to evaluate the bladder's function and efficiency in pediatric and adult patients with various conditions that may cause incontinence or other voiding dysfunctions.

Urologic nurses also practice in long-term care facilities with patients of all ages. Facilities with older residents may utilize the urologic nurse for continence management programs, while facilities with younger clients may focus on urologic-related disorders caused by neurological or spinal cord pathology. As rehabilitation facilities concentrate on maximizing functional status, urologic nurses are utilized to foster independence in self-management of bladder issues, sexual health, and prevention of co-morbidities.

Urologic nurses provide care in a variety of community-based settings such as community-based clinics, home care, or as independent practitioners. Urologic nurses in these practice settings collaborate with community members and lead patient education efforts; organize/staff events for patient screening for urologic cancers; and help patients remain in their homes by providing assistance or education/instruction for self-management of urologic issues. They have collaborated with other health care professionals and community partners in conducting community-based research (Lajiness, Wolfert, Hall, Sampselle, & Diokno, 2007; Palmer & Newman, 2006).

Finally, urologic nurses may combine practice with a faculty position in a nursing or medical academic setting. Nurse educators provide the foundation to prepare associate, baccalaureate, master's, and doctorally prepared nurses in using critical thinking skills, engaging in clinical research, and disseminating their findings to improve practice and patient outcomes. Nurse faculty may lead or collaborate with an interprofessional team in academic health centers and hospital settings to conduct clinical research. Urologic nurses, whose primary role is practice, are involved in education through providing preceptored experiences to nursing students and other health professionals and in continuing education activities. They may also be involved in research through collaboration and coordination with physicians and other health care professionals, or they may be engaged in leading their own research or quality improvement projects.

Differentiation of Registered Nurse and Advanced Practice Registered Nurse Roles In Urologic Nursing

Urologic RNs work in a variety of multidisciplinary and interdisciplinary settings and focus their practice on health promotion, health maintenance, and prevention of illness across the lifespan on individuals, families, and populations who are at risk for developing or presently have urological disorders. The urologic nurse collaborates and serves as an important communicator with other members of the health care team as well as the family, significant others, and the community to implement continuity of care. Urologic nurses act as a patient advocate, assisting the patient seeking information, assuring the patient has the opportunity to make informed decisions for treatment choices, and promoting the maximal level of patient-desired independence. The urologic RN provides and assists in the care of patients undergoing procedures including cystoscopy, prostate biopsy, circumcision, urodynamics, and vasectomy. They are experts in the education of patients and other health care professionals in catheter care, insertion, and the prevention of catheter-associated infections. They convey compassionate, supporting care in the case of the patient with bladder cancer while delivering intravesical chemotherapeutic agents. The urologic nurse may also function in the role of nurse manager, researcher, or educator to assure patient safety and appropriate delivery of care.

The advanced practice registered nurse (APRN) possesses advanced education in physiology/pathophysiology, health assessment, pharmacology, and higher-level clinical skills to manage the individual patient's health care needs. These skills include but are not limited to: providing safe, evidence-based and cost-effective health care; assessment, diagnosis, and management of the patient's health status, including the use and prescription of pharmacologic and non-pharmacologic interventions; monitoring and evaluating the patient's response to treatment, including pharmacologic and non-pharmacologic interventions; and teaching patients and family members to manage complex health problems. APRNs focus on health promotion, disease prevention, early intervention, counseling, and health education for urologic patients and their families across the lifespan (SUNA, 2010). APRNs working in urology health care settings are at the forefront of improving access and managing chronic urologic conditions in a wide range of environments, including independent practices and academic environments (Qaullich, 2011).

Kleier (2009) conducted an exploratory modified two-round Delphi survey of urologic APRNs who were members of SUNA to identify the procedural competencies and job functions unique to the role of the APRN specializing in the care of urologic patients. The implications from this survey inform potential employers as to how urologic APRNs can be used to maximize their practice by providing high-quality, cost-effective care as well as inform continuing nursing education providers of the types of programs that would be most beneficial for urologic APRNs (Kleier, 2009). The American Academy of Nurse Practitioners provides a summary of studies performed between 1981 and 2010 that describe the cost effectiveness of care provided by APRNs by increasing access to health care and overall productivity of their collaborating physicians' practice (Quallich, 2011).

The role of APRNs working exclusively in urology settings appears to be expanding and evolving. A survey was developed and conducted to describe the varied practice settings, tasks, and skills in which APRNs working in the urology setting are employed. Although the sample size was a small, convenience sample of APRNs, the survey demonstrated the role of the APRN blends nursing and medical management, representing clinicians who are ideally positioned to manage many chronic nonoperative urologic conditions, especially those who benefit from a more holistic, patient-centered approach (Quallich, 2011). These advanced practice roles may include but are not limited to primary care provider, consultant, educator, researcher, and administrator in a variety of practice settings.

Professional Education and Development for Registered Nurses and Advanced Practice Registered Nurses

Urologic Registered Nurse

Urologic registered nurses are educationally prepared as generalists in the art and science of nursing upon graduation from an approved school of nursing at the diploma, associate, baccalaureate, master's, or doctoral level. Schools of nursing prepare RNs using a curriculum of general anatomy, physiology, and pathophysiology of the urogenital tract (kidneys, ureters, bladder/urethra, prostate, testes, penis, scrotum), and address nursing management of common urological conditions (urinary incontinence, urinary retention, and urinary catheter-related complications). The urologic RN is educated with the goal of helping individuals and groups attain, maintain, and restore health whenever possible in order to achieve the highest quality of life. In addition to basic educational preparation, understanding the fundamental principles of embryologic development affecting the genitourinary system is necessary to manage care for the pediatric, adult, and elder populations. The foundation of the urologic RN begins with formal education, is broadened through clinical practice, and is grounded by evidence-based research. Compassionate, effective communication and respect are the hallmarks of the urologic nurse due to the sensitive nature of urologic health issues.

There are no formal academic educational programs that exist to prepare RNs in the specialty of urologic nursing. The evolution of urologic nursing specialty training is reliant on individual study, work experience, and on-the-job training. Workplace continuing education and other urology-focused continuing educational programs further the opportunity for professional development in urologic nursing. Professional development courses address other relevant topics as psychosocial needs, quality-of-life issues, support for devastating disease processes, diagnoses, outcomes, and quality improvement projects that translate evidence into clinical practice. Urologic RNs are responsible for the design, administration, and evaluation of professional role development in accordance with the framework established by state nurse practice acts, nursing scope of practice, and organizational standards of care.

Registered nurses interested in advancing their knowledge of or specializing in the field of urology obtain continuing education through resources offered through local, national, and international level courses or conferences. The Society of Urologic Nurses and Associates offers continuing nursing education (CNE) through programs conducted by local chapters, as well as an annual national conference and annual symposium. Nurses attending these conferences have the option of following sub-specialty tracks in urodynamics, pediatric urology, ambulatory care, operating room, or advanced practice. SUNA has an extensive online library that offers audio/visual access to previous conference materials/presentations. SUNA publishes a peer-reviewed professional journal, several clinical practice guidelines, guideline manuals for nursing practice in urodynamics, operating room, telephone triage, and a certification review manual. SUNA has recognized the need for a urologic nursing core curriculum and the project is currently in development.

Urologic RNs bring experience, competence, and the best available evidence and research to care of the patient with urologic conditions. Urologic RNs promote behavioral changes and teach self-care and preventative health care techniques to improve patient outcomes. The Certification Board of Urology Nurses and Associates (CBUNA) acknowledges this specialized knowledge and experience through a rigorous certification process.

Advanced Practice Registered Nurse

Advanced practice registered nurses are clinicians who have completed an accredited or approved APRN program, have obtained a master's or doctoral degree preparing them for a role as a nurse practitioner (NP) or clinical nurse specialist (CNS), have passed a national certification examination for the APRN role, and are registered or licensed by a state board of nursing and recognized as an APRN. The APRN receives additional specialized clinical training and skills beyond their RN preparation. APRNs may also achieve certification in their role specialty.

APRNs demonstrate a greater depth and breadth of theoretical and evidence-based knowledge, a greater synthesis of data, increased complexity of skills and interventions, and significant role autonomy in the field of urologic nursing. CBUNA acknowledges the specialized knowledge and experience of APRNs in urology and offers that level of specialty certification.

The APRN collaborates with, consults with, and serves as liaison to other health care professionals in the field of urology. Advanced practice registered nurses have come to the forefront as primary providers for individuals with urinary incontinence. A survey by Jacobs, Wyman, Rowell, and Smith (1998) indicated most have received no formal urologic training in this area, but a graduate curriculum has since been developed (Rogalski, 2005). APRNs demonstrate a continued commitment to the field of urologic nursing through advocacy and accountability to their profession; community and civic participation; and professional leadership and membership in the Society of Urologic Nurses and Associates, the professional organization responsible for education and excellence in the clinical practice of urologic nurses.

Description of Certification Opportunities

SUNA promotes certification opportunities. CBUNA is the governing body for certification in urologic nursing. Certification promotes standards of nursing care vital to public interest, provides growth and advancement in nursing practice, enhances individual achievement and the individual's sense of professionalism, and promotes a commitment to quality in the delivery of care to the public. The certification test offers an objective measure of the nurse's specialty knowledge and experience in the urologic nursing care of patients and provides evidence of specialty practice (Quallich, 2011). The certification process and eligibility criteria can be found on the SUNA Web site (www.suna.org). Other certifications, such as wound, ostomy, and continence nurses (CWOCN) and peri-operative registered nurses (CNOR), may also be obtained.

Evolution of Urologic Nursing Practice and SUNA

Urologic nursing has continually evolved over the last 40 years. In 1968, Alice Morel, a registered nurse, spearheaded a meeting of those interested in improving education for allied health professionals caring for patients with urological problems. The Urological Nurses Association (UNA) was formed in 1969, and over the next 2 years, many educational and organizational efforts occurred throughout the United States. This included significant collaborative work between early UNA leaders and physician advocates who were members of the American Urological Association (AUA). In 1970, the first scientific program for urologic allied health professionals was sponsored by the AUA in conjunction with their annual meeting.

Rapid growth and development of the UNA occurred over the next decade. This included a change in the name of the organization to the American Urological Association Allied (AUAA). Annual scientific meetings granting continuing education credits were held under the umbrella of the AUA during its annual meeting. Member recruitment with formation of local AUAA chapters, development of written practice guidelines and organizational bylaws, and a standardized certification process were initiated. AUAA's first official newsletter, *Uro-Gram,* was published in 1973 and by 1979, 993 individuals were members of the AUAA.

The 1980s began with publication of the AUAA's first journal (*AUAA Journal*) which within less than 10 years received recognition in the International Nursing Index, was granted a trademark and ISSN number, and in 1988, was renamed *Urologic Nursing. Urologic Nursing* is a peer-reviewed journal that is recognized internationally and has been adopted by the Urology Nurses of Canada as its official journal. AUAA membership surged to over 2,000 members, and attendance at local and regional meetings and workshops, as well as the annual national meeting, continued to grow. Specialty interest groups were formed to support networking and provide specific venues for information sharing among members, and a Core Curriculum was developed. During this time, the AUAA's relationship with the AUA continued to evolve, in addition to involvement with other significant organizations (such as the Nursing Organization Liaison Forum) and industry. These relationships were developed and strengthened, and AUAA leaders conducted a long-range planning meeting.

As the field of urologic nursing continued to grow, AUAA members recognized the need for expanded and more diverse educational opportunities. The 1990s included the addition of an urodynamics workshop, a second national conference (held independent of the AUA meeting and focused on urinary continence), and movement of the annual meeting to a venue and time separate from the AUA annual meeting. Two additional significant changes occurred during this decade: (1) a national health care marketing, communications, publishing, and management firm was selected to provide comprehensive management services to AUAA; and (2) AUAA members voted to change the name of the organization to Society of Urologic Nurses and Associates (SUNA).

Advances in urologic nursing practice supported and led by SUNA have continued into the 21st century. Research and scholarships have long been a focus and part of SUNA's mission, and in 2003 and 2005 respectively the Young Investigator's Research Program and Experienced Investigator's Research Program were launched to provide funding for urologic nursing research. In 2006, the SUNA Foundation was created to improve urologic nursing care via support for nursing research, scholarships, and educational endeavors. SUNA currently provides more than 2,700 members access to legislative information and actively pursues avenues for contributing to national and international quality patient care. SUNA's success is evidenced by well-attended annual conferences and the increasing number of members certified by CBUNA. SUNA leaders are core members of the Global Alliance of Urology Nurses, an alliance of international urologic nursing organizations to promote shared knowledge and networking opportunities.

Current Issues and Trends in Health Care Affecting Urologic Nursing

Issues and trends intersect across nursing specialties, including urologic nursing. As the practice of nursing evolves, a critical understanding of the issues and trends in nursing is necessary.

In 2005, the Centers for Medicare and Medicaid Services (CMS) introduced F-Tag 315, which has made urinary incontinence a major focus and quality indicator in the long-term care setting. Main points of the directive are to minimize indwelling catheter and incontinence pad use and to preserve dignity for residents. Facilities were required to educate staff and residents and to develop programs for individualized treatment of urinary issues. In 2008, CMS brought attention to the issue of hospital-acquired catheter-associated urinary tract infections (CAUTIs). Hospitals were required to reevaluate their policies regarding catheter care and use. Multiple antibiotic-resistant organisms are increasing in our health care facilities and as a result there has been improvement in discussion and awareness in treating asymptomatic bacteriuria in catheterized patients. Education of medical professionals is needed to prevent treatment of bacterial colonization versus true infection, thereby minimizing the overuse of antibiotics. SUNA responded to this need by developing a clinical guideline on CAUTIs for health care providers and disseminating it to members via the SUNA web site.

Incontinence briefs, urinary catheters and medications for overactive bladder, benign prostatic hyperplasia, erectile dysfunction, as well as low testosterone are prominently advertised through television, newspapers, magazines, and the World Wide Web. While some of these portrayals of urinary dysfunction are simplistic, the advertisements are exposing the issues as being commonplace and encouraging individuals to seek treatment. On the other hand, such advertisements may also lead patients to have unrealistic expectations of treatment options for their specific condition. Health care consumers often rely on urologic nursing expertise to explain and interpret the multitude of information and advertisements available.

Hospitals and private practice facilities are also using advertising to promote their delivery of advanced medical and surgical services, especially minimally invasive procedures, including robotics, to attract patients to their facilities.

As our knowledge base evolves, changes in protocols occur. Long-established guidelines for routine prostate specific antigen screening for prostate cancer have recently been challenged, and it is the responsibility of urology professionals to educate patients on any recommended changes in their preventative care routine. As another example, innovations in corrective surgery for stress urinary incontinence and pelvic organ prolapse using minimally invasive surgery with transvaginal placement of surgical mesh has become controversial. Initial results were promising, as the mesh is effective in correcting prolapse, but many patient complications have developed causing the U.S. Food and Drug Administration to issue public health notices with user-reporting requirements. The urologic nurse must continue to monitor evolving practice guidelines, demonstrate patient advocacy, guide and counsel patients related to appropriate decision making, and promote quality outcomes.

Research: Impacts Care, Innovations in Technology

Innovations in technology require an expanding knowledge base for the urologic nurse regarding the care and use of equipment and the education and care of patients undergoing highly technical procedures (robotics and minimally invasive surgery). Patients are treated with a variety of new procedures for bladder control such as botulinum toxin type A (Botox®) injected into the bladder wall, an implantable sacral neuromodulation device for continuous treatment, and percutaneous tibial stimulation therapy for intermittent treatment. Specially trained urologic nurses conduct the programming and application of these neuromodulation treatment devices. Advances in detecting birth defects while the child is in the womb have opened the door for new surgical procedures to correct the defect on the neonate soon after birth. Many formerly complex open pediatric and adult surgeries are performed laparoscopically on an outpatient basis. The urologic nurse develops new competencies or skill sets to render care to the patient and caregivers for safe, optimal outcomes. The urologic nurse may be part of a specialized surgical team who assemble, connect, and calibrate a robotic surgical system for patients undergoing minimally invasive, robotic-assisted laparoscopic surgery.

Electronic medical records, electronic health records, and personal health records are used to improve patient care by facilitating electronic recording, storing, and retrieval of information related to patient care. The urologic nurse may even perform an exam at an off-site clinic in consultation with an urologist utilizing telemedicine conferencing. Nurses and other providers of care must develop and expand computer competencies. Many academic settings offer advanced degrees in informatics to help nurses better navigate the technological environment.

The research work of urologic nurses provides a foundation for answering clinical practice questions. Urologic nurses are in a prime position to develop research studies to answer questions about urologic nursing care and to disseminate findings. A general research session is held at SUNA's Annual Conferences to highlight urologic research and provide attendees with differences that are being made through research. Dissemination stimulates learning, enhances knowledge acquisition, and supports evidence-based clinical decisions. Urologic nurses read and evaluate research and improve patient outcomes by incorporating research-based clinical practice guidelines and evidence-based research findings into practice. Specialty organizations, such as SUNA, help support research and evidence-based practice by providing research grants and forming committees to develop and update clinical guidelines and establish competencies for best practice.

Evidence-Based Practice

Urologic nursing is evidence based. For this reason, it is imperative that research into patient diseases, assessment, treatments, and outcomes continue. The research must be age, culture, race, and gender inclusive to meet the needs of diverse populations. SUNA and other professional organizations work together to develop and continually update best practice and specialty clinical practice guidelines. The Rosswurm and Larrabee (1999) model is a systematic process for adapting existing medical evidence-based practice to a focus on nursing phenomena. The six phases of the model fit with the integration of new knowledge into the development of a urologic nursing protocol or practice change. CBUNA utilizes Patricia Benner's Nursing Theory Model as it looks at novice to expert practices.

Professional and Patient Education

Urologic nurses are actively involved in education of patients, lay caregivers and family members, and other health professionals on topics central to urologic nursing. For example, strategies for infusing urologic content into undergraduate and graduate nursing education have been suggested (Bradway & Cacchione, 2010; Jirovec, Wyman, & Wells, 1998), and two specific examples educators have used in teaching undergraduate nursing students include a focus on helping the students identify their own biases (LeCroy, 2009) and a course assignment highlighting the "lived experience" of wearing absorbent products as a management strategy for urinary incontinence (Karlowicz & Palmer, 2006). Evidence-based, clinical practice guidelines have been developed by SUNA on topics including acute urinary retention, male/female catheterization, and catheter-associated urinary tract infection. SUNA also supports a wide variety of continuing education offerings via local, regional, and national conferences, online Webinars, and publications, including articles in every issue of *Urologic Nursing*.

Urologic Nursing is the official publication of both SUNA and the Urology Nurses of Canada. Contributing authors from multiple health disciplines and from around the world reflect the global and interprofessional influence and esteem of the journal. *Urologic Nursing* serves as a vehicle for timely dissemination of peer-reviewed research and clinically relevant, evidence-based practice manuscripts, clinical case studies, continuing education offerings, and position pieces focused on a wide variety of genitourinary conditions that occur across the lifespan. SUNA members rely on *Urologic Nursing* as a primary educational resource, for professional development opportunities, and as an important benefit of SUNA membership. At least one issue per year is devoted to a special topic relevant to urologic nurses; for example, recent special issues have included informatics, advanced practice nursing, and reducing health disparities and inequalities. During the last decade, the frequency of publication and page count has consistently increased, the ratio of original research articles to review articles and citation of *Urologic Nursing* articles has increased, and a number of new columns have been developed and supported including one focused on the basic tenants of qualitative and quantitative research as they relate to urologic nursing as well as a followup regular column (in almost every issue since 2006) focused on "Translating Evidence into Practice."

SUNA's Annual Symposium and Annual Conference offer an urodynamics training course and advanced urologic practice track for RNs and APRNs desiring to further their knowledge and maintain competencies in their respective practices. The SUNA Web site also has a forum where urologic clinicians have the opportunity to post questions or practice issues for advice and comment from other urologic professionals. Urologic nurses look to SUNA to be the definitive source for urologic nursing education.

There are published guidelines available for teaching patients and family members about urologic care (Zurakowski, Taylor, & Bradway, 2006) and SUNA also makes available a wide variety of detailed patient fact sheets that can be used by urologic nurses in any clinical setting. Urologic nurses utilize innovative techniques and resources to teach self-management skills such as intermittent self-catheterization for patients who need to maintain continence. This need may be due to congenital conditions in children, spinal cord injury in young adults, or age-related changes such as urinary retention in older adults. Teaching self-management skills, such as pessary care in women with pelvic organ prolapse, and Kegel exercises for men and women seeking to restore and maintain continence, can provide a physical and psychological benefit to patients across the lifespan.

Health Care Reform

Access to quality health care is a national issue. People are living longer with multiple chronic diseases, therefore requiring more health care dollars. Given the current health care system, many people face the challenge of being uninsured or underinsured and may not be receiving necessary ongoing health care. Health care reform must focus on primary care and prevention as well as assisting patients with self-management of chronic diseases. SUNA, a member organization of the Nursing Community (a collective of national professional nursing organizations, http://www.thenursingcommunity.org/), supports health care reform issues intended to improve quality care, reduce health care costs, and increase health care access.

Because of the supply-heavy nature of urologic patient care, urologic nurses are also in a unique position to lead the health care team in developing responsible materials management and cost-containment policies. In addition, as health care policies promote the growth and expansion of community-based primary care sites, urologic nurses can be utilized to educate primary care nurses and physicians in best practice for initial assessment and treatment of uncomplicated urologic conditions. Community-based clinics will also require health care professionals to work within a variety of cultural settings. Urologic nurses, as specialized health care professionals, are well suited to provide support and education to culturally and racially diverse populations facing a variety of urologic issues.

Nurses enjoy professional growth and improvement in patient care by advocating for reform of health policies, and lobbying for funding from legislative agencies to promote nursing education, practice, and retention. Urologic nurses can best advocate for patients by participating on legislative committees, writing and publishing scholarly articles focused on issues affecting urologic nurses and patients, and by obtaining professional urologic certification that ensures a prescribed level of competency in the field of urologic nursing.

Challenges to Urologic Nursing

The demand for health care services with an aging population is increasing in the midst of a national nursing shortage. The nursing workforce as a whole is aging and it is difficult to recruit new nurses into the field and retain experienced clinicians. There is a parallel shortage of nursing faculty, further complicating the nursing shortage. Many potential nursing students are turned away from nursing programs due to the shortage of qualified nurse faculty. The Nursing Community actively lobbies for adequate funding for nursing school faculty education as well as funding for government-sponsored nursing scholarship programs.

Nursing Education. Nursing education programs address pathophysiology of the genitourinary system and instruct students in urology-specific competencies for mechanical tasks and procedures such as catheter insertion and bladder irrigation, but deal little with other aspects of urologic nursing. There is, for instance, little instruction provided specific to the overall picture of urologic nursing, the social impact of urologic issues such as incontinence, and the preventative measures health care consumers can take for urologic cancers. Formal educational programs specific to urologic issues are few in comparison to other nursing specialties. There is little reimbursement for specialty nursing education; therefore, it is important for current urologic nurses to identify and mentor nurses from other disciplines who identify an interest or intent to practice as urologic nurses. There is a need for increased funding for urologic nursing education, research, and practice. SUNA has developed brochures to promote the field of urologic nursing specialty.

Professional Development Resources. A global economic downturn, changes to the national health care system, and ever-decreasing reimbursement for specialty services have all led to a decrease in the ability of hospitals and clinics to provide financial support for their staff to attend professional development and CNE offerings. In response, hospitals and clinics have begun offering more on-site education through "Lunch and Learn" classes, on-line continuing education, and utilization of content experts within their own staff. While such on-site learning does not allow for the same networking opportunities as does attending a national conference, it can provide ongoing, accessible information to keep nurses current on delivery of specialty care in their work environments. Professional organizations, such as SUNA, can fill the gap in networking opportunities by facilitating online discussion groups, offering educational Webinars, and using social networking sites to encourage contact between members. CNE is particularly relevant for urologic nurses as the specialty moves from a mainly surgical specialty, to more of a medical-surgical specialty, and the nurses are required to have a broader understanding of co-morbid chronic conditions and their effect on the genitourinary system. As technology advances, urologic nurses must continue to stay current on treatment options, devices, and procedures being offered in the hospital and outpatient settings.

Limitations of Practice. The APRN's roles in the urologic care setting are highly variable. The procedures and activities APRNs are performing cannot be clearly defined due to variations in licensing boards which are governed by regulations and statutes determined by each state. Because of the variation in state regulations regarding the APRN scope of practice, the role of the APRN (nurse practitioner or clinical nurse specialist) is often poorly understood by health care providers, health care consumers, and state regulatory bodies. This has led to restrictions in prescriptive authority, limitations in scope of practice, poor reimbursement for services, and decreased ability for the APRN to practice independently. Urologic APRNs recognize the need to work toward standardization of APRN scope of practice from state to state to address these issues. SUNA is assisting in the endeavor by providing advanced training and developing training guidelines to help APRNs who are asked to perform higher-level procedures. Training APRNs in what were once considered exclusively physician-performed procedures becomes even more important as the number of physicians in full-time practice decreases. Gaines and Quallich (2011) explain that as the physician population ages, and their number of hours worked per week decreases, there will be greater opportunity for NPs with appropriate training to fill gaps in service. Loughlin (2011) alludes to this same phenomenon, but also references how the dearth of urologists in suburban and rural locales limits patient access to urology specialty care. APRNs must take the lead in efforts to ensure their expanded procedural responsibilities are performed safely and effectively.

Cultural and Social Barriers. Purnell and Paulanka (2003) identify cultural competence as "awareness, sensitivity, and transcultural knowledge that permits the culturally congruent care" (p. 4). The intercultural environments nurses work in require them to have the ability and skill to work with culturally and linguistically diverse individuals (Fitzgerald, Williamson, Russell, & Manor, 2005). Being culturally incompetent may result in a loss of opportunity and support for one's decision-making process (Fitzgerald et al., 2005).

Much of the practice of urology deals with issues that are socially and culturally inhibiting such as incontinence and erectile dysfunction in the adult population, or bedwetting in the pediatric population. Nurses of both genders and from various cultures must assist patients with sensitive issues in a culturally competent manner to promote honest discussions about their urologic concerns to improve quality of life. Self-reflection, being open to learning and understanding personal bias or prejudices, will enable the nurse to develop a greater comfort in the ability to communicate with patients and families regarding such sensitive urologic issues. Providing language interpreters and multi-lingual patient education materials are essential as caregivers work toward optimizing the patient's understanding of their situation. Assessment of culturally specific concerns must be performed with regard to recommended diagnostic testing, physical examination, and treatment options.

Summary

Urologic nurses play an essential role in health care. This document, *Urologic Nursing: Scope and Standards of Practice*, provides a comprehensive resource that highlights the mission and evolution of the Society of Urologic Nurses and Associates, and defines and describes the scope of practice, educational preparation, certification, and practice environment/population focus of the urologic RN and APRN. As a dynamic document, current issues and trends are also noted, including those impacting research, evidence-based practice, education, and health care reform. Current challenges to urologic nursing are also described. A commitment to urologic nursing requires that nurses remain involved in continuous professional education and development opportunities, be accountable for strengthening individual practice through a variety of practice settings, as well as maintain membership and support of professional associations such as SUNA. Urologic nursing will continue to strengthen formalized training and education programs for the specialty. Urologic nurses must remain active in legislative initiatives that address nursing education, research, and practice as well as recruitment and retention. Urologic nursing will continue to provide leadership in evidence-based practice and research in order to continue to improve the safety and quality care of individuals for whom they provide care.

STANDARDS OF UROLOGIC NURSING PRACTICE

The public has a right to expect registered nurses to demonstrate professional competence throughout their careers. The RN is individually responsible and accountable for maintaining professional competence. It is the nursing profession's responsibility to shape and guide any process for assuring nurse competence. Regulatory agencies define minimal standards of competence to protect the public. The employer is responsible and accountable to provide a practice environment conducive to competent practice. Assurance of competence is the shared responsibility of the profession, individual nurses, professional organizations, credentialing and certification entities, regulatory agencies, employers, and other key stakeholders (ANA, 2008). In the practice of nursing, competence can be defined, measured, and evaluated. No single evaluation method or tool can guarantee competence. Competence is situational and dynamic; it is both an outcome and an ongoing process. Context determines what competencies are necessary.

The *Standards of Urologic Nursing Practice* are authoritative statements of the duties all urologic nurses are expected to perform competently. The Standards of Practice describe a competent level of nursing care as demonstrated by the critical thinking model known as the nursing process. The nursing process includes the components of assessment, diagnosis, outcomes identification, planning, implementation, and evaluation. Accordingly, the nursing process encompasses significant actions taken by RNs and forms the foundation of the nurse's decision making.

The *Standards of Professional Performance* may be utilized as evidence of care, with the understanding that application of the standards is context dependent; are subject to change with the dynamics of the nursing profession as new patterns of professional practice are developed and accepted by the nursing profession and the public; and are subject to formal, periodic review and revision. The competencies that accompany each standard may be evidence of compliance with the corresponding standard. The list of competencies is not exhaustive for a given standard. Whether a particular standard or competency applies depends upon the circumstances.

STANDARD 1. ASSESSMENT

The urologic registered nurse collects comprehensive data pertinent to the health care consumer's health and/or the situation.

Competencies

The urologic registered nurse:
- Collects comprehensive data in a systematic and ongoing process including but not limited to physical, functional, psychosocial, emotional, cognitive, sexual, cultural, age-related, environmental spiritual/transpersonal, and economic assessments with an emphasis on the urological aspects of health.

- Uses appropriate evidence-based assessment techniques, instruments, and tools, such as uroflowmetry, bladder scans, voiding diaries, validated sexual symptom inventory, prostate symptom score questionnaires, and behavioral interventions.
- Synthesizes available data, information, and knowledge relevant to the situation to identify patterns and variances.
- Prioritizes data collection activities based on the health care consumer's immediate condition, or anticipated needs of the health care consumer or situation.
- Elicits health care consumer values, preferences, expressed needs, and their knowledge of the health care situation.
- Assesses family dynamics and the degree of family support that may impact health care consumer health and wellness.
- Involves the health care consumer, family, and other health care providers as appropriate, in holistic data collection.
- Identifies barriers (e.g., psychosocial, literacy, financial, cultural) to effective communication and make appropriate adaptations.
- Recognizes impact of personal attitudes, values, and beliefs.
- Documents relevant data in a retrievable format.
- Applies ethical, legal, and privacy guidelines and policies to the collection, maintenance, use, and dissemination of data and information.
- Recognizes health care consumers as the authority on their own health by honoring their care preferences.

Additional Competencies for the APRN
The advanced practice registered nurse:
- Initiates and interprets diagnostic tests and procedures appropriate to the health care consumer's current status especially with a focus on the urologic condition such as benign prostatic hypertrophy, infections, incontinence, urinary calculus, congenital disorders, and genitourinary cancers.
- Performs advanced physical assessment based on health care consumer's history, age, and gender.
- Assesses the effect of interactions among individuals, family, community, and social systems to influence and impact health and wellness.
- Conducts preventive screening procedures based on history, age, and gender.

STANDARD 2. DIAGNOSIS
The urologic registered nurse analyzes the assessment data to determine the diagnoses or issues.

Competencies
The urologic registered nurse:
- Derives diagnoses or issues based on the comprehensive assessment data.
- Validates the diagnoses or issues with the health care consumer, family, and other health care providers when possible and appropriate.

- Documents diagnoses or issues to facilitate the plan of care, provides continuity of care and development of measurable outcomes.
- Uses standardized classification systems and clinical decision support tools, guidelines, electronic medical records when available, in identifying diagnoses.
- Identifies actual or potential risks to the health care consumer's health and safety or barriers to health, which may include but are not limited to interpersonal, systemic, or environmental circumstances.

Additional Competencies for the APRN
The advanced practice registered nurse:
- Systematically compares and contrasts clinical findings with normal and abnormal variations and developmental events in formulating a differential diagnosis.
- Assists staff to develop and maintain competency in the diagnostic process of urological problems.
- Utilizes complex data and information obtained during interview, examination, and diagnostic processes in identifying diagnoses.
- Identifies needs of the individual, family, and community based on evaluation of data collected.

STANDARD 3. OUTCOMES IDENTIFICATION
The urologic registered nurse identifies expected outcomes for a plan individualized to the health care consumer or the situation.

Competencies
The urologic registered nurse:
- Involves the health care consumer, family, health care providers, and others in formulating expected outcomes when possible and appropriate.
- Derives culturally appropriate expected outcomes from the diagnoses.
- Defines expected outcomes in terms of the health care consumer, health care consumer culture, values, and ethical considerations.
- Documents expected outcomes as measurable goals with a time estimate for attainment.
- Considers associated risks, benefits, costs, and current scientific evidence, course of illness, health care consumer preferences, and clinical expertise when formulating expected outcomes.
- Develops expected outcomes that facilitate continuity of care.
- Modifies expected outcomes based on changes in the health status of the urologic health care consumer or evaluation of the situation.

Additional Competencies for the APRN
The advanced practice registered nurse:
- Identifies expected outcomes that incorporate scientific evidence and are achievable through implementation of evidence-based practices.
- Determines which outcomes require process interventions from those that require system-level interventions.
- Identifies expected outcomes, taking into consideration cost, clinical effectiveness, health care consumer satisfaction, provider continuity, and consistency of care.

STANDARD 4. PLANNING

The urologic registered nurse develops a plan that prescribes strategies and alternatives to attain expected outcomes.

Competencies

The urologic registered nurse:

- Develops an individualized plan in collaboration with the health care consumer, family, and others considering the person's characteristics or situation, including but not limited to, values, beliefs, spiritual and health practices, preferences, choices, developmental level, coping style, culture, environment, and available technology when appropriate.
- Establishes the plan priorities with the health care consumer, family, and others when appropriate.
- Includes strategies in the individualized plan that address each of the diagnoses or issues. These may include, but are not limited to, promoting and restoring health; preventing injury, illness, or disease; and alleviating suffering and providing supportive care for those who are dying.
- Includes strategies for health and wholeness across the lifespan.
- Provides for continuity in the plan.
- Incorporates an implementation pathway or timeline in the plan.
- Considers the economic impact of the plan on the health care consumer, family, caregivers, or other parties affected.
- Integrates current scientific evidence, trends, and research.
- Utilizes the plan to provide direction to other members of the health care team.
- Defines the plan to reflect current statutes, rules and regulations, and standards.
- Modifies the plan based on the ongoing assessment of the health care consumer's response and other outcome indicators.
- Documents the plan in a manner that uses standardized language or recognized terminology.
- Explores practice settings and safe space and time for the nurse and health care consumer to explore suggested, potential, and alternative options.

Additional Competencies for the APRN

The advanced practice registered nurse:

- Identifies assessment strategies, diagnostic strategies, and therapeutic interventions that reflect current evidence, including data, research, literature, and expert clinical knowledge.
- Selects or designs strategies to meet the multifaceted needs of complex health care consumers.
- Leads the design and development of interprofessional processes to address the identified diagnosis or issue.
- Actively participates in the development and continuous improvement of systems that support the planning process.
- Includes the synthesis of health care consumer's values and beliefs regarding nursing and medical therapies in the plan of care.

STANDARD 5. IMPLEMENTATION

The urologic registered nurse implements the identified plan.

Competencies

The urologic registered nurse:
- Partners with the person/family/significant other/caregiver and other health care providers to implement the plan in a timely, safe, realistic, caring, and non-prejudicial manner.
- Promotes the health care consumer's capacity for the optimal level of participation and problem solving in his/her health care while honoring the person's choices.
- Applies appropriate knowledge of major health problems and cultural diversity in implementing the plan of care.
- Applies available health care technologies to maximize access and optimal outcomes for health care consumers.
- Utilizes available health care technology to measure, record, and retrieve health care consumer data, implement the nursing process, and enhance nursing practice.
- Utilizes evidence-based interventions and treatments specific to the diagnosis or problem.
- Utilizes community resources and systems to implement the plan of care.
- Integrates traditional and complementary health care practices as appropriate.
- Provides holistic care that addresses the needs of diverse populations across the lifespan.
- Advocates for health care that is sensitive to the needs of health care consumers, with particular emphasis on the needs of diverse populations.
- Documents implementation and any modifications, changes, or omissions of the identified plan of care.
- Collaborates with health care providers from diverse backgrounds to implement and integrate the plan of care.
- Implements the plan in a timely manner in accordance with patient safety goals.
- Accommodates for different styles of communication used by health care consumers, families, and health care providers.

Additional Competencies for the APRN

The advanced practice registered nurse:
- Facilitates utilization of systems, organizations, and community resources to implement the plan.
- Supports collaboration with nursing colleagues and other providers to implement the plan.
- Assumes responsibility for a safe and efficient implementation of the plan.
- Uses advanced communication skills to promote relationships between nurses and health care consumers to provide a context for open discussion of the health care consumer's experiences, and to improve health care consumer's outcomes.
- Actively participates in the development and continuous improvement of systems that support the implementation of the plan of care.
- Incorporates new knowledge and strategies to initiate change in nursing care practices if desired outcomes are not achieved.

STANDARD 5A. COORDINATION OF CARE

The urologic registered nurse coordinates care delivery.

Competencies

The urologic registered nurse:
- Documents the coordination of care.
- Communicates with the health care consumer, family, and system during transitions in care.
- Assists the health care consumer in identifying options for alternative care.
- Organizes the components of the plan of care.
- Manages health care consumers' care in order to maximize independence and quality of life.
- Advocates for the delivery of dignified and humane care by the entire inter-professional team.

Additional Competencies for the APRN

The advanced practice registered nurse:
- Provides leadership in the coordination of inter-professional health care for integrated delivery of health care consumer care services.
- Synthesizes data and information to prescribe necessary system and community support measures, including environmental modifications.

STANDARD 5B. HEALTH TEACHING AND HEALTH PROMOTION

The urologic registered nurse employs strategies to promote health and a safe environment.

Competencies

The urologic registered nurse:
- Provides health teaching that addresses the health care consumer's needs and situations throughout the lifespan. These may include, but are not limited to, healthy lifestyles; risk-reducing behaviors; urologic problems and urologic disorders with treatment regimens; self-care activities; community, Internet, and support groups; environmental, behavioral, and lifestyle changes; medications; diagnostic imaging; surgical intervention; diagnostic testing; risk factors for disease; preventive self-care; health maintenance; death and dying issues; mental health disorders; family dynamics; and sexual and reproductive health.
- Uses health promotion and health teaching methods, which are appropriate to the situation and applicable to the health care consumer's values, beliefs, health practices, developmental level, learning needs, readiness and ability to learn, language preference, spirituality, culture, and socioeconomic status.
- Uses information technologies to communicate health promotion and disease prevention information to the health care consumer in a variety of settings.
- Provides information regarding intended effects and potential adverse effects of proposed therapies with attention to urologic therapies.
- Seeks opportunities for feedback and evaluation of the effectiveness of the strategies used.

Additional Competencies for the APRN
The advanced practice registered nurse:
- Synthesizes empiric evidence on risk behaviors; learning theories, behavioral change theories, motivational theories, epidemiology, and other related theories and frameworks when designing health education information and programs on urologic health.
- Designs evidence-based health information and health care consumer education appropriate to the health care consumer's developmental level, learning needs, readiness to learn, and cultural values and beliefs to include urologic conditions.
- Provides anticipatory guidance to individuals, families, groups, and communities to promote health and prevent or reduce the risk of urologic health problems.
- Engages consumer alliances and advocacy groups, as appropriate, in health teaching and health promotion activities related to urologic health.
- Evaluates health information resources, such as the Internet, in the field of urology for accuracy, readability, and comprehensibility to help the health care consumer access quality urologic health information.
- Conducts personalized health teaching and counseling considering comparative effectiveness research recommendations.

STANDARD 5C. CONSULTATION
The advanced practice registered nurse provides consultation to influence the identified plan, provide treatment, enhance the abilities of others, and effect change.

Competencies
The advanced practice registered nurse:
- Synthesizes clinical data, theoretical frameworks, and evidence when providing consultation on urological care.
- Facilitates the effectiveness of a consultation by involving the health care consumer, family, significant other, and stakeholders in decision-making and negotiating role responsibilities.
- Communicates consultation recommendations.

STANDARD 5D. PRESCRIPTIVE AUTHORITY AND TREATMENT
The advanced practice registered nurse uses prescriptive authority, procedures, referrals, treatments, and therapies in accordance with state and federal laws and regulations.

Competencies
The advanced practice registered nurse:
- Prescribes evidence-based treatments, therapies, and procedures considering the health care consumer's comprehensive health care needs.
- Prescribes pharmacologic agents based on a current knowledge of pharmacology and physiology.

- Prescribes specific pharmacological agents or treatments based on clinical indicators, the health care consumer's status and needs, and the results of diagnostic and laboratory tests.
- Prescribes and provides urologic treatment based on clinical assessment.
- Evaluates therapeutic and potential adverse effects of pharmacological and non-pharmacological treatments.
- Provides health care consumers with information about intended effects and potential adverse effects of proposed prescriptive therapies.
- Provides information about costs, alternative treatments, and procedures, as appropriate.
- Evaluates and incorporates complementary and alternative therapies into education and practice.

STANDARD 6. EVALUATION

The urologic registered nurse evaluates progress toward attainment of outcomes.

Competencies

The urologic registered nurse:
- Conducts a systematic, ongoing and criteria-based evaluation of the outcomes in relation to the structures and processes prescribed by the plan of care and the indicated timeline.
- Collaborates with the health care consumer, family, and significant others involved in the care or situation in the evaluation process.
- Evaluates, in partnership with the health care consumer, the effectiveness of the planned strategies in relation to health care consumer's responses, and the attainment of the expected outcomes.
- Uses ongoing assessment data to revise the diagnoses, outcomes, the plan, and the implementation as needed.
- Participates in assessing and assuring the responsible and appropriate use of interventions in order to minimize unwarranted or unwanted treatment and health care consumer suffering.
- Disseminates the results to the health care consumer and others involved in the care or situation, as appropriate, in accordance with state and federal regulations.
- Documents the results of the evaluation.

Additional Competencies for the APRN

The advanced practice registered nurse:
- Evaluates the accuracy of the diagnosis and effectiveness of the interventions and other variables in relationship to the health care consumer's attainment of expected outcomes.
- Synthesizes the results of the evaluation to determine the effect of the plan on the health care consumer, family, groups, communities, and institutions.
- Adapts the plan of care for the trajectory of treatment according to evaluation of the response.
- Uses the results of the evaluation to make or recommend process or structural change including policy, procedure, or protocol revision, as appropriate.

STANDARDS OF PROFESSIONAL PERFORMANCE

The *Standards of Professional Performance* describe a competent level of behavior in the professional role, including activities related to ethics, education, evidence-based practice and research, quality of practice, communication, leadership, collaboration, professional practice evaluation, resource utilization, and environmental health. All registered nurses are expected to engage in professional role activities, including leadership, appropriate to their education and position.

STANDARD 7. ETHICS
The urologic registered nurse practices ethically.

Competencies
The urologic registered nurse:
- Uses *Code of Ethics for Nurses with Interpretive Statements* (ANA, 2001b) to guide practice.
- Delivers care in a manner that preserves and protects health care consumer autonomy, dignity, rights, values, and beliefs.
- Upholds health care consumer confidentiality within legal and regulatory boundaries.
- Takes appropriate action regarding instances of illegal, unethical, or inappropriate behavior that can endanger or jeopardize the best interests of the health care consumer or situation.
- Assists health care consumer in self-determination and informed decision making.
- Maintains a therapeutic and professional health care consumer-nurse relationship with appropriate professional role boundaries.
- Contributes to resolving ethical issues involving health care consumers, colleagues, community groups, systems, and other stakeholders in care of urologic health care consumers.
- Speaks up when appropriate to question health care practice when necessary for safety and quality improvement.
- Advocates for equitable health care consumer care.
- Recognizes the centrality of the health care consumer, family, and significant others as core members of any health care team.

Additional Competencies for the APRN
The advanced practice registered nurse:
- Participates in inter-professional teams that address ethical risks, benefits, and outcomes.
- Provides information on the risks, benefits, and outcomes of health care regimens to allow informed decision making by the health care consumer, including informed consent and informed refusal.

STANDARD 8. EDUCATION

The urologic registered nurse attains knowledge and competence that reflect current nursing practice.

Competencies

The urologic registered nurse:
- Participates in ongoing educational activities related to appropriate knowledge bases and professional issues.
- Demonstrates a commitment to lifelong learning through self-reflection and inquiry to address learning and personal growth needs.
- Seeks experiences that reflect current practice to improve knowledge, skills, abilities, and judgment in clinical practice or role performance.
- Acquires knowledge and skills appropriate to the role of the urology nurse and the care needs of the urologic health care consumer.
- Seeks formal and independent learning experiences to develop and maintain clinical and professional skills, and knowledge with an emphasis on urologic nursing.
- Identifies learning needs based on nursing knowledge, the various roles the nurse may assume, and the changing needs of the population.
- Participates in formal or informal consultations to address issues in nursing practice as an application of education and knowledge base.
- Shares educational findings, experiences, and ideas with peers.
- Contributes to a work environment that is conducive to the education of health care professionals.
- Maintains professional records that document evidence of competency and lifelong learning.
- Attains knowledge of professional practice standards, guidelines, relevant statutes, rules, and regulations regarding nursing practice.

Additional Competencies for the APRN

The advanced practice registered nurse:
- Uses current research findings and other evidence to expand clinical knowledge, skills, abilities, and judgment to enhance role performance and increase knowledge of professional issues.
- Serves as a resource to educate nurses and other groups on the subject of urologic care and management.

STANDARD 9. EVIDENCE-BASED PRACTICE AND RESEARCH

The urologic registered nurse integrates evidence and research findings into practice.

Competencies

The urologic registered nurse:
- Utilizes current evidence-based nursing knowledge, including research findings, to guide practice.

- Incorporates evidence when initiating changes in nursing practice.
- Participates, as appropriate to education level and position, in the development of evidence-based practice through research activities including identifying problems specific to urologic nursing practice and health care consumer care, conducting research, data gathering, critically analyzing and interpreting research for application to practice, serving on a formal committee or program of research, incorporating research as a basis for learning, basing policies, procedures, and standards of practice in health care consumer care on research findings.
- Shares personal or third-party research findings with colleagues and peers.

Additional Competencies for the APRN
The advanced practice registered nurse:
- Promotes a climate of research and clinical inquiry.
- Disseminates research findings through activities such as presentations, publications, consultation, and journal clubs.
- Contributes to nursing knowledge by conducting or synthesizing research and other evidence that discovers, examines, and evaluates current practice, knowledge, theories, criteria, and creative approaches to improve health care outcomes.
- Collaborates with other health care professionals and health care consumers to identify areas of research.
- Supports translational research in the field of urology.

STANDARD 10. QUALITY OF PRACTICE
The urologic registered nurse contributes to quality nursing practice.

Competencies
The urologic registered nurse:
- Demonstrates quality by documenting the application of the nursing process in a responsible, accountable, and ethical manner.
- Uses creativity and innovation in nursing practice to improve delivery of nursing care to urology health care consumers.
- Participates in quality improvement activities. Such activities may include:
  - Identifies problems in day-to-day work routines in order to correct process inefficiencies.
  - Implements processes to remove or decrease barriers within organizational systems.
  - Analyzes factors related to quality, safety, and effectiveness.
  - Analyzes quality data to identify opportunities for improving nursing practice.
  - Analyzes organizational systems for barriers to quality health care consumer outcomes.
  - Identifies aspects of practice important for quality monitoring.
  - Uses indicators developed to monitor quality, safety, and effectiveness of nursing practice.
  - Collects data to monitor quality and effectiveness of nursing practice.
  - Formulates recommendations to improve nursing practice or outcomes.
  - Implements activities to enhance the quality of urology nursing practice.

- Develops, implements, and evaluates policies, procedures, and/or guidelines to improve the quality of urology nursing practice.
- Participates in and/or leads inter-professional teams to evaluate clinical care or health services.
- Participates in and/or leads efforts to minimize costs and unnecessary duplication of services.
- Obtains and maintains professional certification if available in the area of expertise.

Additional Competencies for the APRN
The advanced practice registered nurse:
- Provides leadership in the design, implementation, and evaluation of quality improvement activities.
- Designs innovations to effect change in practice and improve health outcomes.
- Evaluates the practice environment and quality of nursing care rendered in relation to existing evidence.
- Identifies opportunities for the generation and use of research and evidence.
- Obtains and maintains professional certification in the area of expertise.
- Uses the results of quality improvement activities to initiate changes in nursing practice and in the health care delivery system.

STANDARD 11. COMMUNICATION
The urologic registered nurse communicates effectively in a variety of formats in all areas of practice.

Competencies
The urologic registered nurse:
- Assesses communication format preferences of health care consumers, families, and colleagues.
- Assesses own communication skills in encounters with health care consumers, families, and colleagues.
- Seeks continuous improvement of own communication and conflict resolution skills.
- Conveys information to health care consumers, families, the inter-professional team, and others in communication formats that promote accuracy.
- Questions the rationale supporting care processes and decisions when they do not appear to be in the best interest of the health care consumer.
- Discloses observations or concerns related to hazards and errors in care or the practice environment to the appropriate level.
- Maintains communication with other providers to minimize risks associated with transfers and transition in care delivery.
- Contributes own professional perspective in discussions with the inter-professional team.

STANDARD 12. LEADERSHIP

The urologic registered nurse demonstrates leadership in the professional practice setting and the profession.

Competencies

The urologic registered nurse:
- Oversees the nursing care given by others while retaining accountability for the quality of care given to urology health care consumers.
- Abides by the vision, the associated goals, and the plan to implement and measure progress of an individual health care consumer or progress within the context of the health care organization.
- Demonstrates a commitment to continuous, lifelong learning and education for self and other members of the health care team.
- Mentors others to advance nursing practice, the profession, and to achieve quality health care.
- Treats health care consumers, colleagues, and other members of the health care team with respect, trust, and dignity.
- Develops communication and conflict resolution skills.
- Participates in professional organizations, including the Society of Urologic Nurses and Associates.
- Communicates effectively with the health care consumer and colleagues.
- Seeks ways to advance nursing autonomy and accountability.
- Participates in efforts to influence health care policy involving health care consumers and the profession.

Additional Competencies for the APRN

The advanced practice registered nurse:
- Influences decision-making bodies to improve and influence health care policy involving the professional practice environment and health care consumer outcomes.
- Provides direction to enhance the effectiveness of the inter-professional team.
- Mentors colleagues in the acquisition of clinical knowledge, skills, abilities, and judgment.
- Models expert practice to inter-professional team members and health care consumers.
- Promotes advanced practice nursing and role development by interpreting the APRN role for health care consumers, families, and others.

STANDARD 13. COLLABORATION

The urologic registered nurse collaborates with the health care consumer, family, and others in the conduct of nursing practice.

Competencies
The urologic registered nurse:
- Partners with others to effect changes and generate positive outcomes by sharing knowledge of the health care consumer and/or situation with others.
- Communicates with the health care consumer, family, and health care providers regarding health care consumer care and the nurse's role in the provision of that care.
- Promotes conflict management and engagement.
- Participates in building consensus or resolving conflicts in the context of health care consumer care.
- Applies group process and negotiation techniques with health care consumers and colleagues.
- Adheres to standards and applicable codes of conduct that govern behavior among peers and colleagues to create a work environment of cooperation, respect, and trust.
- Cooperates in creating a documented plan focused on outcomes and decisions that reflect communication with the health care consumer, families, and others involved in the health care consumer's care.
- Engages in teamwork and team-building processes.

Additional Competencies for the APRN
The advanced practice registered nurse:
- Partners with other disciplines to enhance health care consumer outcomes through inter-professional activities such as education, consultation, management, technological development, or research opportunities.
- Invites the contribution of the health care consumer, family, and interdisciplinary team in achieving optimal outcomes of care.
- Leads in establishing, improving, and sustaining collaborative relationships to achieve safe, quality health care for the health care consumer.
- Documents plan of care communications, rationales for plan of care changes, and collaborative discussions to improve health care consumer outcomes.

STANDARD 14. PROFESSIONAL PRACTICE EVALUATION

The urologic registered nurse evaluates one's own nursing practice in relation to professional practice standards and guidelines, relevant statues, rules, and regulations.

Competencies
The urologic registered nurse:
- Provides age and developmentally appropriate care in a culturally and ethnically sensitive manner.

- Engages in self-evaluation of practice on an ongoing basis, identifying areas of strength as well as areas in which professional development would be beneficial.
- Obtains informal feedback regarding one's own practice from health care consumers, peers, professional colleagues, and others.
- Participates in peer review as appropriate.
- Takes action to achieve goals identified during the evaluation process.
- Provides the evidence for practice decisions and actions as part of the informal and formal evaluation processes.
- Interacts with peers and colleagues to enhance one's own professional nursing practice or role performance.
- Provides peers with formal and informal constructive feedback regarding their practice or role performance.

Additional Competencies for the APRN
The advanced practice registered nurse:
- Engages in formal evaluation process seeking feedback regarding one's own practice from health care consumers, peers, professional colleagues, and others.

STANDARD 15. RESOURCE UTILIZATION
The urologic registered nurse utilizes appropriate resources to plan and provide nursing services that are safe, effective, and financially responsible.

Competencies
The urologic registered nurse:
- Assesses individual health care consumer care needs and resources available to achieve desired outcomes.
- Identifies health care consumer care needs, potential for harm, complexity of the task, and desired outcomes when considering resource allocation.
- Delegates elements of care to appropriate health care workers in accordance with any applicable legal or policy parameters or principles.
- Identifies the evidence when evaluating resources.
- Advocates for resources, including technology, that enhance nursing practice.
- Modifies practice when necessary to promote a positive interface between health care consumers, health care providers, and technology.
- Assists the health care consumer and family in identifying and securing appropriate and available services to address needs across the health care continuum.
- Assists the health care consumer and family in factoring costs, risks, and benefits in decisions concerning treatment and care.

Additional Competencies for the APRN
The advanced practice registered nurse:
- Utilizes organizational and community resources to formulate inter-professional plans of care.
- Develops innovative solutions utilizing the best resources for health care consumer care problems, without sacrificing quality of care.
- Develops evaluation strategies that demonstrate cost benefit, cost effectiveness, and efficiency factors associated with nursing practice.

STANDARD 16. ENVIRONMENTAL HEALTH
The urologic registered nurse practices in an environmentally safe and healthy manner.

Competencies
The urologic registered nurse:
- Attains knowledge of environmental health concepts, such as implementation of environmental health strategies.
- Promotes a practice environment that reduces environmental health risks for workers and health care consumers.
- Assesses the practice environment for factors such as sound, odor, noise, and light that negatively affect health.
- Communicates environmental health risks and exposure-reduction strategies to health care consumers, families, colleagues, and communities.
- Participates in strategies to promote healthy communities.
- Advocates for the judicious and appropriate use of products used in health care.
- Utilizes scientific evidence to determine if a product or treatment is a potential environmental threat.

Additional Competencies for the APRN
The advanced practice registered nurse:
- Creates partnerships that promote sustainable environmental health policies and conditions.
- Analyzes the impact of social, political, and economic influences on the environment and human health exposures.
- Critically evaluates the manner in which environmental health issues are presented by the popular media.
- Advocates for implementation of environmental principles for nursing practice.
- Supports nurses in advocating for and implementing environmental principles in nursing practice.

References

American Nurses Association (ANA). (2001). *Code of ethics for nurses with interpretive statements.* Washington, DC: American Nurses Publishing.

American Nurses Association (ANA). (2008). Professional role competence position statement. In *Nursing: Scope and standards of practice* (2nd ed.). Silver Spring, MD: Nursebooks.org

American Nurses Association (ANA). (2010a). *Nursing: Scope and standards of practice* (2nd ed.). Silver Spring, MD: Nursebooks.org

American Nurses Association (ANA). (2010b). *Nursing's social policy statement: The essence of the profession.* Silver Spring, MD: Nursebooks.org

Bradway, C., & Cacchione, P. (2010). Teaching strategies for assessing and managing urinary incontinence in older adults. *Journal of Gerontological Nursing, 36*(7), 18-26.

Fitzgerald, M., Williamson, P., Russell, C., & Manor, D. (2005). Doubling the clock of (in)competence in client/therapist interactions. *Medical Anthropology Quarterly, 19*(3), 331-347.

Gaines, K.K., & Quallich, S. (2011). Toward advances in practice. *Urologic Nursing, 31*(6), 325-326.

Gray, M., & Moore, K. (2009). *Urologic disorders: Adult and pediatric care.* St. Louis, MO: Mosby, Inc.

Jacobs, M., Wyman, J.F., Rowell, P., & Smith, D.A. (1998). Continence nurses: A survey of who they are and what they do. *Urologic Nursing, 18*(1), 13-20.

Jirovec, M., Wyman, J.F., & Wells, T.J. (1998). Educational competencies for urinary incontinence. Guidelines for curriculum development. *Image, 30,* 375-378.

Karlowicz, K.A., & Palmer, K.L. (2006). Engendering student empathy for disabled clients with urinary incontinence through experiential learning. *Urologic Nursing, 26*(5), 373-378.

Kleier, J.A. (2009). Procedure competencies and job functions of the urologic advanced practice nurse. *Urologic Nursing, 29*(2), 112-117.

Lajiness, M.J., Wolfert, C., Hall, S., Sampselle, C., & Diokno, A.C. (2007). Group session teaching of behavioral modification program for urinary incontinence: Establishing the teachers. *Urologic Nursing, 27*(2), 124-127.

LeCroy, C.A. (2009). The perception of urinary incontinence. *Urologic Nursing, 29*(3), 145.

Loughlin, K.R. (2001). Urologists on a tightrope: Have we lost our balance? *Urology, 77*(3), 525-532.

Nursing Community. (n.d.). Retrieved from www.thenursingcommunity.org

Palmer M.H., & Newman, D.K. (2006). Bladder control educational needs of older adults. *Journal of Gerontological Nursing, 32*(1), 28-32.

Purnell, L., & Paulanka, B. (Eds.). (2003). *Transcultural health care* (2nd ed.). Philadelphia, PA: F.A. Davis Company.

Quallich, S.A. (2011). A survey evaluating the current role of the nurse practitioner in urology. *Urologic Nursing, 31*(6), 328, 330-336.

Rogalski, N.M. (2005). A graduate nursing curriculum for the evaluation and management of urinary incontinence. *Educational Gerontology, 31,* 139-159.

Rosswurm, M.A., & Larrabee, J.H. (1999). A model for change to evidence-based practice. *Image Journal Nursing Scholarship, 31*(4), 317-322.

Society of Urologic Nurses and Associates (SUNA). (2010). *APRN fact sheet.* Pitman, NJ: Author.

Zurakowski, T., Taylor, M., & Bradway, C. (2006). Effective teaching strategies for the older adult with urological concerns. *Urologic Nursing, 26*(5), 355-360.

Additional Readings

APRN Consensus Work Group & the National Council of State Boards of Nursing APRN Advisory Committee. (2008). *Consensus model for APRN regulation: Licensure, accreditation, certification and education.* Retrieved from http://www.aacn.nche.edu/education-resources/APRNReport.pdf

Cancer Statistics, 2011. (2011). *CA: A Cancer Journal for Clinicians, 61*(4), 212-236.

Karlowicz, K.A. (Ed.). (1995). *Urologic nursing: Principles and practice.* Philadelphia, PA: W.B. Saunders.

Society of Urologic Nurses and Associates. (1997). *Scope and standards of urologic nursing practice.* Pitman, NJ: Author.

Society of Urologic Nurses and Associates. (1999). *Scope and standards of advanced urologic nursing practice.* Pitman, NJ: Author.

Todd, B.A., Resnick, A., Stuhlemmer, R., Morris, J.B., & Mullen, J. (2004). Challenges of the 80-hour resident work rules: Collaboration between surgeons and nonphysician practitioners. *Surgical Clinics of North America, 84*(6), 1573-1586.